POSTPARTUM DIET

FOR NOVICES

Enriched Recipes, Foods, Meal Plan & Procedures For Boosting Energy, Body Nourishment, Weight Loss And Vibrant Health For New Mothers

DR. MATEO GABRIEL

DISCLAIMER

The information in this book is only meant to be used for general reading. In any way, the author and publisher do not promise or represent that the information in this work is full, correct, reliable, appropriate, or available. This includes any warranties that are expressed or implied. Because of this, you should only rely on this material at your own risk.

This book is not meant to replace professional help. If you have any questions about a subject, you should always get help from a qualified expert. The author and distributor of this book are not responsible for how the information in it is used or abused.

The author's thoughts and feelings are shown in this book. They do not necessarily represent the official policy or stance of any other person, group, employer, or business.

Any third-party material that you can get to through this book is not endorsed or backed by the author or publisher.

The information in this book is correct at the time it was published, after all possible checks. However, the author and distributor are not responsible for any loss, damage, or inconvenience that may be caused by mistakes or omissions.

TABLE OF CONTENTS

CHAPTER ONE

INTRODUCTION TO POSTPARTUM DIET

Often referred to as the fourth trimester, the postpartum period is a crucial time in a woman's path toward parenting. The body is going through a period of tremendous physical and emotional changes as it recovers from pregnancy and childbirth. Nutrition is one essential component of postpartum care that requires careful consideration. To promote the mother's physical recovery, meet the needs of breastfeeding, and enhance her general well-being, postpartum nutrition is essential. To support optimum healing, energy levels, and mental well-being during this time, a sophisticated grasp of nutritional requirements is necessary.

THE SIGNIFICANCE OF POSTPARTUM NUTRITION

Postpartum nutrition is essential for both mother and baby development and is not only a question of what to cook. During the postpartum period, the body's nutritional needs change significantly, necessitating careful consideration while making food decisions. Restoring depleted nutritional stores, such as iron and calcium, that may have been used during pregnancy requires adequate eating during this time. Furthermore, the recovery of tissues affected during childbirth, such as the uterus and perineum, is closely associated with postpartum nutrition.

Beyond healing physically, the postpartum diet plays a major role in mental wellness. Hormonal changes during this time can affect one's mood, energy level, and emotional health in general. A balanced diet that provides both macro- and micronutrients can be quite helpful in reducing these swings and promoting the mental well being of mothers. A comprehensive approach to postpartum treatment must address nutritional demands in light of anticipated difficulties including anxiety and sadness.

SUMMARY OF POSTPARTUM DIET OBJECTIVES

The postpartum diet objectives cover a wide range of topics to meet the various demands of both the mother and the baby. First and foremost, it's critical to maintain a healthy calorie intake, particularly for nursing moms who need extra energy to sustain the production of milk. It is imperative to maintain a balanced intake of macronutrients, such as proteins, lipids, and carbs, to fulfill energy requirements and supply the fundamental building blocks needed for tissue healing and repair.

Consuming micronutrients is similarly important because there is typically a greater need for certain vitamins and minerals during the postpartum phase. For example, iron is necessary to prevent postpartum anemia and to restore maternal storage. Consuming enough calcium promotes bone health, which is advantageous for the growing child as well as the mother. Furthermore, introducing meals high in omega-3 fatty acids helps the nursing infant's cognitive development.

Although it's often disregarded, hydration is a crucial component of postpartum nutrition. Adequate hydration promotes tissue healing, is necessary for lactation, and helps avoid frequent postpartum problems like constipation. When you take into account the stress of taking care of a baby and the possibility of sleep deprivation, it becomes even more important for mothers to drink enough water.

Comprehensive care for new mothers requires an understanding of the profound effects of postpartum nutrition on both physical and mental health. A customized approach to food choices is necessary during the special and delicate postpartum period, as meeting specific nutritional goals is crucial for the best possible recovery and overall well-being.

CHAPTER TWO

COMPREHENDING POSTPARTUM DIET

NUTRITIONAL NEEDS DURING POSTPARTUM

The postpartum period, commonly referred to as the fourth trimester, is a key time for new moms as they recuperate from childbirth and adapt to the duties of caring for a newborn. During this era, attention to nutrition was vital to promote the physical and emotional well-being of both the mother and the infant. Postpartum nutritional needs encompass a combination of factors, including replenishing nutrient stores depleted during pregnancy and childbirth, supporting breastfeeding if applicable, and promoting overall recovery.

Adequate caloric intake is essential to meet the increased energy demands associated with breastfeeding, especially for mothers who choose to nurse their infants. Nutrient-dense foods, such as fruits, vegetables, whole grains, and lean proteins, play a pivotal role in replenishing essential vitamins and minerals. Hydration is equally important, as breastfeeding can lead to increased fluid loss. Proper hydration aids in milk production and supports the mother's overall recovery.

In addition to macronutrients, postpartum nutrition should focus on micronutrients crucial for recovery and maintaining optimal health. Iron and calcium, for instance, are vital for replenishing stores depleted during pregnancy and childbirth, promoting bone health, and preventing anemia. Omega-3 fatty acids, found in fish and flaxseeds, are essential for both brain development in the baby and cognitive function in the mother.

HORMONAL CHANGES AND THEIR IMPACT ON DIET

The postpartum period is marked by significant hormonal fluctuations as a woman's body transitions from pregnancy to the postpartum state. Hormones such as estrogen, progesterone, and prolactin play key roles in orchestrating various physiological changes, impacting appetite, metabolism, and nutrient utilization. Understanding these hormonal shifts is crucial in tailoring a diet that supports both physical recovery and emotional well-being.

Prolactin, the hormone responsible for milk production, can increase appetite in breastfeeding mothers. This heightened appetite is a natural response to the increased energy demands of lactation. However, mothers need to make nutritious food choices to meet these demands without resorting to empty-calorie foods. Including nutrient-dense snacks and meals is crucial in ensuring that the increased caloric intake aligns with the nutritional needs of both the mother and the breastfeeding baby.

Estrogen and progesterone levels, which dramatically drop after childbirth, can influence mood and energy levels. A well-balanced diet rich in complex carbohydrates, proteins, and healthy fats can help stabilize blood sugar levels, providing a sustained source of energy and positively impacting mood. Incorporating foods that support serotonin production, such as whole grains and lean proteins, can contribute to a sense of well-being during this emotionally challenging period.

COMMON NUTRIENT DEFICIENCIES IN POSTPARTUM WOMEN

Despite the emphasis on postpartum nutrition, many women may experience common nutrient deficiencies during this period. Iron deficiency anemia is prevalent, as iron stores are often depleted during pregnancy and childbirth. Including iron-rich foods such as lean meats, beans, and leafy greens can help replenish iron stores and prevent fatigue and weakness.

Calcium deficiency is another concern, particularly for breastfeeding mothers, as calcium is crucial for both bone health and milk production. Dairy products, fortified plant-based milk, and leafy green vegetables are excellent sources of calcium that can address this deficiency.

Omega-3 fatty acids, essential for brain development in infants, are commonly lacking in postpartum diets. Incorporating fatty fish, flaxseeds, and walnuts can help bridge this nutritional gap. Vitamin D deficiency is also prevalent, and sunlight exposure and dietary sources like fortified foods and supplements may be recommended.

Understanding and addressing the nutritional needs of postpartum women involves a holistic approach that considers the physical and hormonal changes occurring during this unique phase.

A well-balanced diet, rich in essential nutrients, plays a pivotal role in supporting recovery, promoting emotional well-being, and ensuring the health and vitality of both the mother and her newborn.

CHAPTER THREE

BUILDING A FOUNDATION: THE BASICS OF A POSTPARTUM DIET

BALANCED NUTRITION

A crucial aspect of a postpartum diet is achieving balanced nutrition, which involves obtaining the right proportions of macronutrients and micronutrients. Macronutrients, including carbohydrates, proteins, and fats, play a pivotal role in providing energy and supporting various physiological functions. Carbohydrates, in the form of whole grains, fruits, and vegetables, contribute to sustained energy levels.

Proteins are essential for tissue repair and muscle recovery, while healthy fats aid in hormone production and absorption of fat-soluble vitamins.

In addition to macronutrients, paying attention to micronutrients is equally important during the postpartum period. Vitamins and minerals such as iron, calcium, vitamin D, and folate are crucial for overall health and the recovery process. Incorporating a diverse range of nutrient-dense foods, including leafy greens, dairy products, and lean proteins, ensures a well-rounded and balanced postpartum diet.

HYDRATION AND ITS IMPORTANCE

Staying adequately hydrated is paramount for postpartum recovery. Hydration plays a crucial role in maintaining bodily functions, supporting breastfeeding mothers, and replenishing fluids lost during labor and delivery. Water is essential for the production of breast milk, aiding digestion, and promoting skin health.

Postpartum women should attempt to consume an ample amount of water throughout the day. Dehydration can contribute to fatigue, headaches, and a decreased milk supply for breastfeeding women. It is vital to heed the body's cues for thirst and make a conscious effort to ingest water-rich meals, such as fruits and vegetables, to boost overall hydration.

INCORPORATING FIBER INTO THE DIET

A postpartum diet should focus on the incorporation of dietary fiber to maintain digestive health and prevent constipation, a major issue during this period. Fiber-rich foods, such as whole grains, fruits, vegetables, and legumes, aid in regulating bowel movements and contribute to a sensation of fullness, which can be beneficial for managing postpartum weight.

Additionally, integrating fiber into the diet encourages the growth of good gut bacteria, promoting a healthy microbiome. This is particularly significant for postpartum women as it can positively benefit both their health and the development of the infant's gut microbiome.

Developing a good foundation for postpartum nutrition entails taking a balanced strategy that covers macronutrients, micronutrients, appropriate hydration, and fiber intake.

CHAPTER FOUR

MEAL PLANNING FOR NEW MOTHERS

CREATING A POSTPARTUM MEAL PLAN

Creating a postpartum meal plan is a vital feature of assisting new mothers during a time when their bodies are recovering and adjusting to the demands of caring for a newborn. The key to a good postpartum meal plan is in its capacity to provide nutritional, well-balanced meals that respond to the individual demands of a new mother.

This involves addressing nutritional requirements for postpartum recovery, lactation, and overall energy levels.

Focusing on nutrient-dense foods that promote lactation and aid in healing is a fundamental idea in creating a postpartum meal plan. This entails including a range of food groups, including whole grains, fruits, vegetables, lean proteins, and healthy fats. Furthermore important for milk production and the healing process is getting enough water.

EASY AND QUICK RECIPES FOR WORKING MOTHERS

Since caring for a baby frequently involves time limits and weariness, postpartum meal plans should prioritize quick and simple meals. For time-pressed mothers, one-pot meals, sheet pan dinners, and slow cooker dishes can be lifesavers as they provide wholesome meals with little work or effort.

With the demands of motherhood, these recipes make it easier for new mothers to prioritize their nutrition because they can be easily put together or cooked in advance.

IDEAS FOR SNACKS TO MAINTAIN ENERGY

Snack options are essential for maintaining energy levels throughout the day, in addition to main meals. New mothers must snack because they can find it difficult to sit down for regular meals. Healthy fats, carbs, and protein are the components of ideal snacks. A handful of trail mix, nut butter on whole grain crackers, or Greek yogurt with berries is a few examples.

These snacks add to the total amount of nutrients required for postpartum recovery in addition to giving a rapid energy boost.

Understanding how important convenience is, it's a good idea to keep healthful snacks readily available in the kitchen. This reduces the tendency to choose less nourishing items when you're tired or hungry.

The postpartum meal plan can be made more pleasurable and fulfilling by including a range of textures and flavors in snacks, which will motivate new mothers to put their nutrition first.

A well-planned postpartum meal plan takes into account the unique nutritional requirements of new moms while also taking nursing, postpartum recuperation, and the difficulties of a hectic schedule into account.

With its emphasis on nutrient-dense foods, simple and quick meals, and healthy snack ideas, the meal plan turns into an invaluable resource for promoting the general health of the mother and her baby.

Making nutrition a priority for self-care is a critical first step toward facilitating a more seamless transition to parenthood during this critical postpartum phase.

CHAPTER FIVE

ESSENTIAL ELEMENTS FOR POSTPARTUM REJUVENATION

IRON AND SOURCES ARE IMPORTANT FOR NEW MOMS

A vital component of postpartum healing, iron helps the body rebuild its reserves following the large blood loss experienced during childbirth. Adoptive mothers frequently feel weak and exhausted, so getting enough iron in their diet is crucial to boosting vitality and general health. Hemoglobin, the protein that carries oxygen in the blood and is essential for the body's postpartum repair, is made up primarily of iron.

New mothers can get their iron from both plant- and animal-based sources. Heme iron, or iron that the body can readily absorb, is abundant in lean meats, poultry, fish, and eggs. Non-heme iron is found in plant-based foods including beans, lentils, fortified cereals, and dark leafy greens. Although it is absorbed less effectively, non-heme iron can nevertheless make a substantial contribution to blood iron levels. It may be advised to take iron supplements, particularly for individuals who are at risk of insufficiency. However, it is imperative to speak with a healthcare provider to ascertain the proper amount.

POSTPARTUM BONE HEALTH AND CALCIUM

Another crucial mineral for postpartum healing is calcium, which primarily supports bone health. The body may use the mother's calcium reserves to assist fetal development throughout pregnancy; therefore, it's critical to make sure the mother replenishes these reserves postpartum and avoids long-term problems like osteoporosis. While nursing, a baby's teeth, and bones are developing with the help of an adequate calcium intake.

Milk, cheese, and yogurt are dairy items that are high in absorbable calcium. They are also great sources of calcium. For people who cannot tolerate lactose or choose not to drink dairy, leafy green vegetables, tofu, and fortified plant-based milk substitutes can be excellent sources of calcium. If food consumption is inadequate, supplements may also be advised; however, as with any supplement, it is crucial to discuss specific needs with a healthcare professional.

OMEGA-3 FATTY ACIDS FOR MOOD AND BRAIN DEVELOPMENT

Omega-3 fatty acids are essential for postpartum healing because they promote the mother's mental health and newborn brain development. These important fatty acids are passed to the fetus throughout pregnancy and lactation, especially docosahexaenoic acid (DHA) and eicosapentaenoic acid (EPA), which are critical components of the brain. Additionally, omega-3s contain anti-inflammatory qualities that may help lessen the symptoms of postpartum depression.

Omega-3s are abundant in fatty fish, including mackerel and salmon, which provide both EPA and DHA. Walnuts, chia seeds, flaxseeds, and algae-based supplements provide plant-based substitutes for fish for individuals who might not eat it. Including these foods in the diet helps the mother's general mood and well-being throughout the taxing postpartum period, in addition to supporting the baby's cognitive development. As always, speaking with a medical expert can assist in figuring out the best dietary or supplement strategy for a certain set of circumstances.

CHAPTER SIX
FOODS TO TAKE AND LEAVE OUT

TOP FOODS TO CONSUME AFTER GIVING BIRTH

New moms need to emphasize foods that promote healing and supply vital nutrients during the delicate postpartum recovery period. Refueling the body with nutrients after childbirth and pregnancy requires incorporating a diet rich in nutrients and well-balanced. Rich in iron and vitamin K, dark leafy vegetables like kale and spinach promote healthy blood coagulation and general energy levels. Fish, poultry, and lentils are examples of foods high in lean protein that aid in energy restoration and muscle regeneration.

Eating foods high in omega-3 fatty acids, such as chia seeds and salmon, is good for your body and mind. Because of their well-known anti-inflammatory qualities, omega-3 fatty acids help to reduce postpartum inflammation and support a positive outlook. Healthy grains such as brown rice and quinoa also offer a wonderful dose of complex carbohydrates that promote general healing and give prolonged energy.

In addition, obtaining the necessary calcium from dairy or fortified plant-based substitutes is crucial for maintaining bone health and preventing postpartum osteoporosis. Foods high in probiotics, such as kefir and yogurt, can improve gut health by facilitating digestion and nutrient absorption. Clear broths, herbal teas, and lots of water should be favored during the postpartum time because they are all equally vital for hydration.

FOODS TO REFRAIN FROM EATING

While eating a healthy diet is crucial, new mothers should also be aware of some products that could impede their body's ability to heal after giving birth. Foods that are highly processed and loaded with additives and preservatives have to be consumed in moderation because they may cause inflammation and upset the hormonal balance. Caffeine overindulgence, which can be found in coffee and other energy drinks, should also be avoided as it can disrupt sleep cycles and dehydrate the body.

Refined sweets and high-fat foods should be avoided as they might cause energy spikes and crashes that can negatively affect one's general well-being. Additionally, to reduce discomfort during the healing phase, foods like beans and cruciferous vegetables that are known to induce gas or bloating should be ingested in moderation. Drinking alcohol should be done with caution since it can interfere with the body's natural healing processes and, if you're nursing, may have an impact on the production of breast milk.

PARTICULAR THINGS TO KEEP IN MIND FOR NURSING MOTHERS

Nutritional considerations for breastfeeding moms go beyond self-healing to benefit their infants' growth and well-being. Maintaining a sufficient calorie intake is essential to satisfy the higher energy needs of nursing. Incorporating a varied range of nutrient-dense foods, such as whole grains, lean proteins, and vibrant fruits and vegetables, guarantees that breast milk contains an important nutrient composition.

Foods high in calcium, like dairy products or fortified substitutes, are still essential for the development of the baby's bones as well as the mother's bones. Flaxseeds and fatty fish are good sources of omega-3 fatty acids, which help develop the baby's brain and eyes. Mothers who are nursing should drink enough water since dehydration can reduce milk production.

Although a lot of foods are acceptable to eat while nursing, certain babies might be allergic to certain things that are passed on through breast milk. Mothers should watch their baby's reactions and be aware of potential allergens like dairy, nuts, and gluten.

CHAPTER SEVEN
MANAGING POSTPARTUM WEIGHT
HEALTHY METHODS FOR LOSING WEIGHT

After giving birth, maintaining a healthy weight is a gradual process that calls for a variety of thoughtful tactics, including a balanced diet, consistent exercise, and constructive self-care routines. Effective weight reduction techniques are essential for new moms to lose excess weight while maintaining their dietary requirements.

A diet rich in nutrients and well-balanced is essential for managing weight after childbirth. Making whole foods a priority, such as fruits, vegetables, lean meats, and whole grains, gives the mother and the infant (if nursing) the vitamins and minerals they need. Including a range of nutrients promotes general health and facilitates healing. Portion control is key, and restrictive diets should be avoided since they can impair energy and interfere with the body's natural healing process.

EXERCISE AND HEALING AFTER CHILDBIRTH

A crucial element of weight management and postpartum recuperation is exercise. Walking, swimming, and postpartum-friendly workout regimens are a few examples of activities that might help enhance cardiovascular health, elevate mood, and facilitate weight loss. To avoid damage and allow the body to heal, it is essential to approach exercise patiently and increase intensity gradually. To make sure that a postpartum fitness regimen fits with each person's unique health demands and recovery process, speaking with a healthcare provider before beginning is advised.

SELF-CARE AND BODY IMAGE

In addition to being physical, postpartum recovery involves emotional healing as well, and dealing with body image issues is essential to the process. New moms frequently experience excessive stress as a result of the need to live up to societal norms. Good body image requires accepting changes in the body and engaging in self-compassion practices. It can be helpful to surround oneself with a network of friends, relatives, or other mothers who can offer understanding and support during this time of transition.

Postpartum weight management is greatly influenced by self-care, which includes both physical and mental health. Finding time for relaxation, meditating, and getting enough sleep can all have a great effect on general health and help with weight management. A more sustainable approach to weight loss is made possible by striking a balance between the demands of motherhood and self-care, which also promotes resilience and a sense of equilibrium.

Postpartum weight management calls for a comprehensive strategy that takes into account safe weight reduction techniques, sensible exercise regimens, and self-care routines that promote a positive body image. By adopting these ideas, new moms can focus on their physical and mental health throughout the postpartum phase, leading to a more sustainable and healthy way of living.

CHAPTER EIGHT

TAKING CARE OF TYPICAL POSTPARTUM PROBLEMS WITH DIET

OVERCOMING FATIGUE AND INCREASING VITALITY

Deep exhaustion is a common postpartum symptom as new moms adjust to the duties of caring for a newborn and experience physical and hormonal changes. Dietary management of fatigue is essential for general health. Eating a range of fruits and vegetables, whole grains, lean meats, and other nutrient-dense foods can give you a steady supply of energy. Foods high in iron, like as leafy greens and lean meats are essential in preventing postpartum anemia, which is a major cause of exhaustion. Additionally, one of the most important things you can do to prevent fatigue is to be well-hydrated by drinking enough water.

FOODS THAT PROMOTE MENTAL WELL-BEING

A mother's mental health is particularly vulnerable during the postpartum phase, and nutrition is important for promoting emotional health. Omega-3 fatty acids, which are present in walnuts and fatty seafood like salmon, have been related to happier moods and may help with postpartum depression symptoms.

Including complex carbs in your diet, such as those found in whole grains and legumes, can help control your serotonin levels and help you feel happier. Dark leafy greens and berries are two examples of meals high in antioxidants that support brain function overall and may help lower oxidative stress.

HANDLING POSTPARTUM DIGESTIVE PROBLEMS

Constipation, bloating, and other digestive problems are sometimes brought on by hormone fluctuations, changed gut motility, and nutritional modifications. Digestive problems are a common postpartum worry. Consuming meals high in fiber, such as fruits, vegetables, and whole grains, can help control bowel movements and stave off constipation. Foods high in probiotics, such as kefir and yogurt, bring good bacteria into the stomach and support a healthy digestive tract. Additionally, staying hydrated is essential for preserving regularity and avoiding dehydration, which can make stomach pain worse. By making these dietary changes gradually, the digestive tract can adjust without experiencing further stress.

Getting through the postpartum phase requires dealing with a variety of emotional and physical difficulties.

CHAPTER NINE

PARTICULAR DIETS AND NUTRITIONAL LIMITATIONS

POSTPARTUM DIETS THAT ARE VEGAN OR VEGETARIAN

Supporting a new mother's health and well-being after giving birth requires postpartum nutrition. It becomes crucial for people who lead vegetarian or vegan lifestyles to make sure their food choices sufficiently satisfy their nutritional needs at this delicate time. Vegan diets go even further and forbid all animal products, including dairy and eggs, in addition to meat, as does a vegetarian diet.

The main goals of a postpartum diet that is well-balanced and vegetarian or vegan should be to gain important nutrients including protein, iron, calcium, vitamin B12, and omega-3 fatty acids. To address potential inadequacies, plant-based protein sources such as beans, tofu, and quinoa can be included in addition to fortified foods or supplements. To guarantee that the mother and child receive enough nutrients for optimum health and development, careful planning is essential.

GLUTEN-FREE FOODS AND ADDITIONAL DIETARY FACTORS

It's critical to follow a gluten-free diet for people who have celiac disease or gluten sensitivity. Wheat, barley, and rye contain the protein gluten, which can cause negative side effects in those with gluten-related conditions. Following a gluten-free diet during the postpartum phase necessitates careful meal selection to avoid unintentional gluten intake.

Individual health problems or preferences may also give rise to additional dietary issues. Certain people may follow ketogenic or low-carb diets, while others may be subject to dietary restrictions related to their culture or religion.

Obtaining advice from medical specialists or trained dietitians is essential to create a customized postpartum diet that meets nutritional requirements and promotes general health.

SENSITIVITIES AND ALLERGIES IN POSTPARTUM DIET

In addition, the postpartum diet needs to include sensitivity and allergy issues that could impact the nursing newborn or the mother. Common allergies including soy, dairy, eggs, and nuts might make some people react negatively. To avoid allergic reactions in both themselves and their babies, moms with known allergies or sensitivities must closely manage the foods they choose.

Women who are nursing their babies should exercise extra caution because some allergens' proteins can enter their breast milk. When an infant has allergies, it may be advised to go through an elimination and reintroduction phase to pinpoint the cause and modify the

Postpartum nutrition is a customized and intricate facet of maternal healthcare. The health and recuperation of the mother and the newborn depend heavily on a well-planned and balanced diet, regardless of whether the mother chooses to live a vegetarian or vegan lifestyle, manages gluten sensitivity, or navigates allergies and sensitivities.

CHAPTER TEN
ESTABLISHING A HELPFUL ENVIRONMENT

INCLUDING THE FAMILY IN POSTPARTUM EATING

Establishing a nurturing atmosphere in the postpartum phase is essential for the health of the mother and the infant. A crucial element of this assistance is integrating the family into the postpartum diet. Family is essential in helping the new mother with both practical and emotional assistance. Encouraging family members to take an active role in organizing and cooking wholesome meals promotes a feeling of solidarity and shared accountability. This engagement helps to reinforce family ties at this pivotal time while also ensuring that the mother gets the nutrition she requires. Involving the family in postpartum nutrition fosters a supportive atmosphere that goes beyond the mother's urgent needs, enhancing the family's general well-being and harmony.

LOOKING FOR EXPERT ADVICE

Creating a supportive postpartum environment also requires seeking professional help. Numerous physical and mental changes that new mothers frequently go through can be rather stressful. Consulting with healthcare experts, such as dietitians, nutritionists, or lactation consultants, offers specialized knowledge and recommendations to meet each person's needs. Experts can provide advice on specific dietary considerations during the postpartum phase, supplementation, and optimal nutritional choices. This helps the mother feel more secure and powerful as she transitions into parenthood by easing her worries and ensuring that she receives evidence-based care. One proactive step in creating a network of support that puts the health and well-being of the mother and the infant first is involving experts in postpartum care.

OBTAINING COMMUNITY ASSISTANCE

Getting support from the community is also essential to creating a loving atmosphere for new mothers. Developing relationships with other parents who are going through comparable circumstances fosters understanding and comradery. Participating in community activities catered to new families, taking parenting classes, or joining online or local support groups can offer a platform for exchanging experiences, getting advice, and forming enduring friendships. The collective wisdom and empathy that develops when people band together to deal with the difficulties and rewards of the postpartum phase is what gives community support its potency. Through proactive pursuit and involvement in communal assistance, recentlyweds can create a support system of like-minded people who foster a feeling of acceptance and joint accountability during their motherhood journey.

Establishing a nurturing atmosphere during the postpartum phase necessitates a diverse strategy that encompasses educating family members about postpartum nutrition, obtaining expert advice, and locating community resources. These related ideas work together to create a comprehensive support network that attends to new moms' social, emotional, and physical needs. Combining these components creates a supportive atmosphere that enhances the health and well-being of the mother and the infant as they travel through the life-changing experience that is postpartum.

CHAPTER ELEVEN

PROLONGED POSTPARTUM DIET

MAKING THE SWITCH TO A HEALTHFUL, SUSTAINABLE DIET

For moms to promote their general well-being in the long-term postpartum period, switching to a sustainable and healthful diet is essential. Developing dietary practices that support immune system function, mental health, and sustained energy becomes critical as they negotiate the demands of parenthood. A varied range of nutrient-dense foods, including whole grains, lean proteins, fruits, vegetables, dairy products, and dairy substitutes, should be included in a balanced diet. Incorporating seasonal and locally obtained produce into meal options emphasizes sustainability, which benefits both individual health and environmental preservation.

Furthermore, adopting a sustainable diet frequently entails consuming fewer packaged and processed foods, which are frequently heavy in added sugars, bad fats, and preservatives. Mothers can maximize their nutrient intake and promote long-term health advantages by choosing whole, minimally processed foods. A sustainable and healthy diet not only provides for a mother's physical needs but also her mental health by promoting her sense of well-being and giving her the energy she needs to take care of her expanding family and everyday chores.

ORGANIZING FOR UPCOMING PREGNANCIES

Planning is crucial for mothers who are considering getting pregnant in the long-term postpartum phase. A key factor in getting the body ready for the demands of a second pregnancy is nutrition. For example, consuming enough folic acid before conception lowers the growing fetus's risk of neural tube abnormalities. For the sake of both the mother and the fetus, it is crucial to maintain adequate amounts of essential minerals like iron, calcium, and vitamin D in later pregnancies.

Mothers can maximize their nutritional status in anticipation of future pregnancies by eating a well-balanced diet that includes a variety of nutrients and taking the needed prenatal supplements, as advised by healthcare professionals. Beyond food restrictions, regular physical activity and keeping a healthy weight improve general well-being and can enhance fertility. Mothers negotiating the shift from postpartum to subsequent pregnancies must seek the guidance and close supervision of healthcare specialists.

THE PART NUTRITION PLAYS IN MOTHERS' AGING

The importance of nutrition in the aging process increases with the age of moms. After giving birth, a woman's life is not over, and it is crucial to think about the long-term effects of food decisions to age well. The need for some nutrients can change as we age, so it's important to make sure you're getting enough of them to keep your bones, brain, and general vigor intact.

Including foods strong in calcium and vitamin D is crucial for maintaining bone health, especially for women who are more susceptible to osteoporosis as they age. Furthermore, walnuts, flaxseeds, and fatty fish—all high in omega-3 fatty acids— may support cognitive function, which is especially important for mothers navigating the aging process. Fruits and vegetables high in antioxidants are essential for boosting the immune system, reducing oxidative stress, and improving skin health.

Postpartum nutrition over the long term is a dynamic and changing component of a mother's life.

www.ingramcontent.com/pod-product-compliance
Lightning Source LLC
Chambersburg PA
CBHW050748260726
48661CB00001B/475